Coming to Terms
with Type 1 Diabetes

One Family's Story of Life After Diagnosis

DEBBIE YOUNG

Coming to Terms with Type 1 Diabetes
One Family's Story of Life After Diagnosis

Copyright © Debbie Young 2014
Foreword © Justin Webb 2014

Published by Hawkesbury Press
First published in digital format 2013
This paperback edition first published 2014
Also available as an ebook

Cover design by SilverWood Books
www.silverwoodbooks.co.uk

Cover image © George Gooding 2014
Used with his kind permission

ISBN: 978-0-9930879-0-5

British Library Cataloguing in Publication Data
A CIP catalogue record for this book is available
from the British Library

PRAISE FOR THIS BOOK

From the medical profession:

"A lovely uplifting little book, full of insight, wit, and practical know-how. I think it will appeal to anyone with Type 1 diabetes and their family. Health professionals would also find it useful. The book is beautifully written. A little treasure as well as a ray of hope."

Dr Carol Cooper, GP, President of the Guild of Health Writers, author, broadcaster & lecturer at Imperial College, London

From parents whose children have Type 1 diabetes:

"An amazing book, very moving, thought provoking and inspiring. Essential reading for anyone who cares for someone with Type 1 diabetes. Raising money for the best of causes to prevent and treat this awful disease."

Louise Arnold

"A great book for parents of children just diagnosed with Type 1 diabetes – identifying with other parents' feelings is just what you need when your child is newly diagnosed."

Lisa Hirst

"An honest account of the emotional journey following a diagnosis and the impact it can have within a family. Debbie takes the tough bits with the positives and writes from the heart."

Jacky Taylor

From other authors:

"A heart-warming, honest account of a mother's shock, acceptance, and ongoing battle after her 3-year-old daughter's diagnosis with Type 1 diabetes. Debbie Young has an amazing way with words, combining heart-breaking moments with inspiration and courage and above all hope... hope for a cure. What an admirable way of raising funds to try and find a cure for this terrible disease."

Liza Perrat, author of Spirit of Lost Angels

"The lightness and freshness in Debbie Young's writing about this unwelcome aspect of her family's life is a symptom of her toughness and will-power. But it's also a symptom of a richly developed sense of proportion and priorities, proactively applied with strong intelligence across the complex landscape of practical logistics and emotional demands that attend this diagnosis.

"Like other major diagnoses (whether physical or mental), this one causes a person's life picture to receive a big gash of unwelcome colour across part of it... but the picture's subject remains that same person in all their other glories, despite that gash... and with the likes of Debbie in the house, those glories succeed in meeting that gash with a straight bat, optimistically re-arraying themselves with clear-eyed pragmatism, sensitivity and humour, so as to carry on engaging with the many fascinations of life, unimpoverished and undaunted."

Rohan Quine, author of The Imagination Thief

"Families of children with diabetes will find comfort in these pages, but even those whose lives have not been touched by this illness – yet – should read this book. Oh, and have a packet of tissues handy when you do."

Joanne Phillips, author of Can't Live Without

CONTENTS

A NOTE FROM JDRF UK

I am so thankful to Debbie for choosing to donate the profits from this special book to JDRF – and for writing with such honesty and emotion, in a way that will provide encouragement and hope to those who are affected by the condition.

Type 1 diabetes affects about 400,000 people in the UK, 29,000 of them children. A child diagnosed with the condition at the age of five faces up to 19,000 injections and 50,000 finger prick blood tests by the time they are 18.

JDRF funds research to cure, treat and prevent Type 1 diabetes. We provide information for children, adults and parents living with the condition, at all stages from diagnosis and beyond. We give a voice to people with Type 1 diabetes and campaign for increased focus on, and funding for, research to find the cure. Internationally, JDRF is the world's leading charitable funder of Type 1 diabetes research. We work with academia, industry and governments to make sure that the research we fund has the greatest possible impact on the lives of people with Type 1 diabetes now and in the future.

With the help of amazing supporters such as Debbie, we will continue to make progress on the journey towards the cure.

Karen Addington
Chief Executive
JDRF UK
www.jdrf.org.uk

JDRF is a registered charity in England and Wales number 295716
and in Scotland number SC040123

FOREWORD
by Justin Webb

It began, for my family, with a car crash in America. My 8-year-old son Sam and I were zooming along in my convertible on Washington's equivalent of the M25 when, just ahead, someone spun off the road.

We were past the scene in a flash; Sam didn't even see it. He looked back when I pointed it out. I think the drivers involved were okay, but we talked about how suddenly life can change. Bad things can happen even when you don't deserve it. Days later, for Sam, they did.

He had been tired for weeks. We had been back to the UK to sort out schools, so we assumed it was jet lag. But that didn't explain his thirst, an amazing, prodigious thirst that would have him gasping for water morning, noon and night. With the thirst came the need to urinate, and at night a bedwetting that we hadn't seen for years.

Three days before Christmas, after a doctor's appointment and a lot of waiting, the verdict was delivered in a room with a rather nice view of the car park. I wasn't even there – I had rushed home to talk to the BBC news desk, thinking life was carrying on as normal.

It was not. For families around Britain and around the world, today and tomorrow, and for every day until a cure is found, a diagnosis of Type 1 diabetes is a life-altering, life-worsening piece of news. Their daily struggle to cope, which begins with that news, can never end. For parents, for the children themselves, all is changed.

Some cope badly and suffer the awful consequences of complications and added misery. But some people have within them (perhaps they did not know it) the strength to fight back, to do something, both for themselves but also for the struggle to find a cure.

This book has been written by someone who is ready and willing and able to fight back, and I commend her for it. Debbie Young has written a moving and personal testimony. I hope it inspires people to support the work of the JDRF. And to salute the pioneers who first helped Type 1 diabetics to stay alive, and nowadays help them to live increasingly normal lives. This is a story that begins with harsh reality but encompasses success as well. It is a story of hope and progress, and one day it must end, in triumph.

Justin Webb
Journalist & Presenter of BBC Radio 4's Today Programme

THE BEGINNING
(10 May 2007)

Like Justin Webb and his family, we're accustomed to living with Type 1 diabetes in our household.

Thirteen years ago, Gordon, now my husband, started to lose weight dramatically. He kept nodding off to sleep during the day, and on waking was desperately thirsty. When I told him it seemed unhealthy to drink a whole litre carton of orange juice, he disagreed.

"Of course it's not unhealthy! I'm full of Vitamin C!"

Nevertheless, he agreed to visit his GP. He knew why I was anxious: unexpected weight loss had been an early symptom of my first husband John's terminal leukaemia. I was terrified that Gordon's diagnosis would be the same.

Gordon's opening gambit to the doctor was: "There's nothing wrong with me, I'm just here to make my girlfriend happy."

A couple of days later, a letter arrived in the post. Gordon was to report to the surgery immediately to begin treatment for diabetes. I was thrilled: it wasn't leukaemia. But it was a lifelong, incurable condition that would radically change Gordon's daily life and health, and, unbeknown to me, our unborn daughter's too. My relief was short-lived.

And so the treatment began – treatment that would never cure his diabetes, just hold it sufficiently in abeyance to keep him alive. The more carefully he managed his condition, the greater chance he would have of averting serious complications in the long term.

Effective management of Type 1 diabetes is harder than it sounds. It's not to be confused with Type 2 diabetes, often associated with being overweight or with lifestyle choices, and in which the body continues to produce insulin but becomes less efficient in using it. In Type 1, the body stops producing insulin completely. The only remedy is to introduce insulin into the body artificially. Unfortunately, taking insulin orally is not an option, because it is a protein which would be broken down in the digestive system. Therefore it must be delivered by another means, either by injection from a hypodermic syringe or from an insulin pump via a cannula (a small needle and tube permanently penetrating the flesh).

Insulin is short-acting, which means that the body's stores need continual replenishment, typically at least four injections every day or a constant drip-feed from a pump. The requirement to either stab yourself repeatedly, every day, with hypodermic needles or to wear a pump 24/7 is not the only factor to make managing Type 1 diabetes unusually demanding. Unlike any other medical condition that I know, Type 1 diabetes requires the patient, rather than a medical professional, to calculate exactly how much insulin to take. This is because the body's need for insulin is affected by many variables which change from day to day and from hour to hour:

- your current blood glucose level (determined by pricking your finger with a lancet to extract a bead of blood for testing)
- the carbohydrate content of what you are about to eat (not just sugar, but any form of carbohydrate, a substance that is present in most staples such as bread, pasta, rice, some fruit and vegetables, and milk)
- the speed at which your planned meal or snack will digest (you must time the administration of the dose to match the rate at which the food will be absorbed)
- how physically active you've been (if you're active enough, your insulin requirement may shrink to nothing, and you may even need to take extra "free carbs" without insulin to prevent a hypo)
- bizarrely enough, the weather (temperature can make a surprising difference to the required dose)
- your age (the action of growth hormones caused by pubertal growth spurts, the menstrual cycle and the menopause can play havoc with the calculations)

Ideally, every person with Type 1 diabetes should know how to calculate their insulin doses, taking all of these variables into account. One seldom takes the same dose twice in succession. Not all people have the skills required – numeracy, planning, confidence – or the motivation to do it day in, day out, with no chance of respite. It is a tiresome, rigorous routine. It makes measuring out a dose of Calpol seem like child's play, (not that you'd trust a child to give themselves Calpol, either). Many struggle constantly to get it right, and many, frankly, get it wrong.

Failure is not a great option, because failure would increase risks of serious long-term health problems: permanent damage to the eyesight, heart, circulatory system and nervous system.

I was soon to realise that Gordon's diagnosis with Type 1 diabetes wasn't such good news after all.

A couple of years later, after our marriage, our only daughter, Laura, was born. She was a lovely, late surprise: I was 43. I couldn't believe my good luck to have such a perfect child. When she was 3, I discovered the catch: she developed Type 1 diabetes. The news hit me with the force of a bereavement, and I went into mourning for the loss of my child's unblemished health.

Intrinsically optimistic, I clutched at straws of comfort:

- It was not leukaemia
- Compared to the children and babies we'd seen on the ward who had life-limiting illnesses, she was relatively well.
- We had caught it at a very early stage: she did not go into DKA (diabetic ketoacidosis), the potentially fatal toxic shock that develops in untreated Type 1 diabetes.
- She hadn't inherited another illness that peppered my husband's family: female cancers passed down through the BRCA gene. (My goodness, how I sobbed with relief when a clear test result came through.)
- She was not Madeleine McCann, who had gone missing the previous week. Laura and Madeleine were only 11 days apart in age and, with blonde bobbed hair and big blue eyes, very similar in appearance. For months afterwards, I expected to be accosted on the street when I was out with Laura by people who thought I'd kidnapped Madeleine. I was relying on the absence of the black flash in Madeleine's right eye to save me from likely arrest.

Even so, I struggled to come to terms with the knowledge that Laura's diagnosis with Type 1 diabetes had changed our lives forever. I knew I had no choice: I had to cope, and I was determined to do so from day one. When the nurse arrived at Laura's hospital bedside to deliver her first ever insulin injection, I volunteered to administer it myself. I knew I had to get on with it. It was the first injection of the rest of our lives.

Next, I sought knowledge. When confronting illness, knowledge is power. I'd discovered that with John's leukaemia. I read voraciously, joined support networks, and took an Open University course called Living with Diabetes.

I adopted as a mantra the advice given by Helen, our wonderful Paediatric Diabetes Specialist Nurse: "Don't let the diabetes rule your life – you rule the diabetes." Another of the many invaluable pieces of advice we received was "Don't blame yourselves". Both Gordon and I were wracked with assumed guilt, because he had Type 1 diabetes himself, and I had several other auto-immune disorders in the same family as Type 1 diabetes: rheumatoid arthritis, vitiligo and hypothyroidism. Being told very clearly that it was not our fault saved us wasting emotional and mental energy on a misplaced sense of guilt.

In time, I began to use my experience to help others. I gave moral support to other parents whose children had been diagnosed, offering a shoulder to cry on, sharing tips that we'd come across (Love Hearts as a cool hypo remedy – who knew?), and, most important of all, I listened. I attended information days run by the Type 1 diabetes charity JDRF (formerly known as the Juvenile Diabetes Research Foundation). These inspirational events demonstrated ingenious developments by hugely creative scientists who were devoting their careers to finding better therapy and a cure.

On these occasions, I realised just how far research and development had come. Earlier generations had to boil up on their kitchen stoves huge glass syringes and needles for their injections. They had crude, unreliable testing methods such as urine tests that only told them what their blood glucose had been a few hours before, rather than at the time of the test, potentially leaving dangerous highs and lows untreated until too late. The first insulin pump would not have been portable for a child: it was the size of an astronaut's backpack.

By contrast, we have the benefit of smart, light, compact single-use needles that make it far easier to give sterile injections. We have simple-to-use electronic testing devices that give accurate results within seconds, allowing for immediate appropriate corrective treatment. We have insulin pumps so small and compact that they're often mistaken for mobile phones. Whenever offered the chance to trade up to the latest therapy, we took it. Switching from multiple daily injections to an insulin pump transformed the quality of life for both Laura and Gordon.

Having come so far, we must be able to go further. To any family affected by Type 1 diabetes, JDRF spells hope. Finding out about their work made me want to raise funds for research. I tried the usual suspects: table-top sales, sponsored walks, sponsored runs. But it wasn't enough. I sought more.

Following the diagnosis of Type 1 diabetes, there are various stages of grief that the whole family must pass through. I knew about grief; I'd been there when I was widowed. When we eventually arrived at the stage of acceptance, we began to reshape our family life accordingly.

It was only at this stage that I started to do what has helped me cope with crises all my life: I wrote about it. Not medical advice – of course not, only qualified professionals should do that, although it's widely acknowledged by doctors and nurses that some patients and their parents become very knowledgeable indeed about the management of Type 1 diabetes – but about my feelings, my hopes and my longing that one day a cure will be found.

I didn't want to write about it often, for fear of boring my friends and losing my audience altogether. Nor did I want to become obsessive or self-pitying, a trap that's very easy to fall into. I just needed to write enough to release the pressure I was feeling, and to do something constructive to raise funds for the search for a cure.

On my personal blog, *www.authordebbieyoung.com*, I published a number of essays about Type 1 diabetes and JDRF. Normally this blog is the preserve of light-hearted posts about whatever takes my butterfly mind's fancy. I hoped that by shoehorning these serious missives in among the usual flippant waffle, they might have more impact. I sought the opposite effect of comic relief. But blog posts, like newspapers, swiftly disappear. Today's newly-published post is tomorrow's virtual fish-and-chip wrapper. I wanted to put my essays to more lasting use. So here they are now, reclaimed from cyberspace and bolted together without the previous frivolous dividers. Publishing them gives me the opportunity to air them before a wider audience while also raising research funds for JDRF and boosting awareness of the charity's important work.

This book was first published as an ebook for World Diabetes Day 2013. It quickly attracted excellent reviews from a wide spectrum of readers, including some groups I hadn't planned to target, e.g. medical professionals.

Producing this new print edition, published to mark World Diabetes Day 2014, will enable me to reach more readers, to help more families, and to gain more support for the JDRF. It will remain in print until a cure is found – because for those affected by Type 1 diabetes, every day is Diabetes Day. And that needs to change.

BIRTHDAY THOUGHTS & DIABETES
(18 January 2010)

What is JDRF? It's a fabulous charity with a global network raising money to find a cure for Type 1 diabetes. This condition was formerly known as juvenile diabetes because it is usually diagnosed in relatively young patients. However, it can strike at any age after birth.

The incurable lifelong illness that is Type 1 diabetes is becoming increasingly common. If untreated, it is certainly fatal. Even with twenty-first century therapies, keeping Type 1 diabetes in check is a constant, relentless struggle. When my small and otherwise perfect daughter Laura was diagnosed with Type 1 diabetes at the age of 3, so began our 24/7 battle with this unpredictable and unruly condition.

Why did Laura get it? No-one knows. Type 1 diabetes is just one of life's lesser lotteries, with a prize no-one ever wants to win.

Asked when starting school at the age of 4 to describe herself in a single word, Laura replied "Diabetic". No child should have to give that answer. Ask me for one word to describe myself and I'd say "Writer". I'm grateful that I have a natural facility with words, but I'd trade that talent tomorrow for a cure for Type 1 diabetes. Today, when I blow out my 50 birthday-cake candles, a cure is what I shall wish for, even though I know that wishing alone won't work.

In the meantime, there is something else I can do to hasten the discovery of a cure: I can use my way with words to raise awareness and funds for JDRF's search for a cure.

DEALING WITH DIAGNOSIS
(9 May 2011)

Thirteen days before Laura's fourth birthday, on 10 May 2007, I took her to the doctor's. There had recently been a heat-wave. She'd been drinking a lot during the hot weather, so it was no surprise that she was also weeing a lot.

When her extraordinary thirst continued after the weather had turned cold, I put it down to a minor urinary infection and booked a routine appointment with our GP. My worst fear was that we'd come away with a course of antibiotics. I wasn't looking forward to having to make her take a course of tablets. If only we'd got off that lightly. Instead, we were immediately dispatched to hospital as an emergency with a diagnosis of Type 1 diabetes.

"Are you in a fit state to drive?" said the GP as I sobbed silently behind Laura's back. "If not, I'll call an ambulance and we'll blue-light you there."

Neither of us was being over-dramatic. Without treatment, Laura could have become critically ill within hours – and dead before she could turn 4.

Type 1 diabetes shows no mercy. It can strike at any age. It strikes at random and without obvious cause. It's not lifestyle related. It's no-one's fault. It's a death sentence if you don't take your insulin. And even if you do, it's a life sentence because you have to keep taking insulin, every day, for the rest of your life.

To help you work out how much insulin to take, you need to test your blood glucose many times a day, pricking your fingers with a lancet to release the required bead of blood. It hurts. It makes a mess. It's no fun at any age. But it beats the only alternative. That would be death, then. Compared to death, having your fingertips permanently flecked with puncture marks is a walk in the park.

Refusing insulin therapy is unthinkable in developed countries, because without it the patient will quickly die. Elsewhere people may not have the choice. Many die, all over the world, because they live in countries too poor to provide insulin therapy.

But there is hope: active research programmes funded by the JDRF and other international organisations are on the verge of finding better ways of managing diabetes. They seek easier means of delivering insulin, less invasive ways of monitoring blood sugar, and therapies to reduce the long-term health risks. One day, with enough funding, they may be able to prevent the disease, to slow down its onset, maybe reverse it, and even find a cure.

As any parent of a child with Type 1 diabetes will tell you, the best way to cope with diagnosis is to hold out hope of a cure.

~ 4 ~

NOT ALL DREAMS ARE IMPOSSIBLE
(14 June 2012)

So I dream of a cure for Type 1 diabetes. Is this an impossible dream? I don't think so.

Clearly I'm not able to make scientific breakthroughs myself: I'm no Marie Curie. But there are incredibly talented, inspired and dedicated scientists in this world who, with enough money to fund their research, will one day find a cure. Of this I am sure. And I defy you to look my lovely daughter Laura in the eye and say you don't care whether or not it's ever found.

Type 1 diabetes is a devastating disease. If you are unfortunate enough to get it, it is likely to strike you in childhood – and if you get it, you've got it for life. There's no known cause or cure. It's a life sentence.

Diagnosed at the age of 3, Laura cannot remember life without this condition. No, she will not grow out of it. Exhibit A: my husband. But Laura is lucky - she gets the treatment she needs.

She's lucky – she has the sterile needles required to safely prick her fingers four or more times a day for her blood tests.

She's lucky – the NHS supplies clean needles or cannulas and the insulin needed to provide her daily injections or infusions.

She's lucky – she has loving parents willing and able to manage her therapy effectively until she's old enough to do it herself.

She's lucky – she's now got an infusion pump with a tube sunk into her flesh 24/7 to deliver her life-saving insulin subcutaneously.

We're lucky – she's brave and uncomplaining by nature.

When anyone thoughtlessly complains that they've got to have a one-off inoculation or blood test, I have to bite my tongue. I want to tell them tersely that they ought to try a few days living with Type 1 diabetes. Laura's a seasoned veteran of the hypodermic needle and the cannula – the plastic tube that must be inserted with a long needle and changed every two days. Her fingertips are pitted with black dots from her multiple daily bloods tests. And no matter how often you stick needles into yourself, it hurts.

I'm not after pity for my family's plight. What I really want is a cure – not just for my darling daughter or husband, but for the generations of children yet to come, all over the world, who will continue to suffer from this wretched disease and, in poor countries, to die until we find a cure. Please help me to help them.

Every penny donated to JDRF brings that cure a little closer.

In the meantime, Laura sends hugs.

ANOTHER NICE MESS FOR LAUREL & LAURA
(13 November 2011)

On the eve of World Diabetes Day 2011, as Laura and I watched one of our boxed set of Laurel and Hardy DVDs, I discovered through my newly acquired pocket guide to their films that the great Stan Laurel was diabetic. I wasn't sure whether he was Type 1 or Type 2 so I gave him the benefit of the doubt and assumed he was Type 1, for companionship.

Laura was delighted to hear the news. Sharing an illness provided a new bond with her comedy hero. Watching the credits earlier, she'd wished aloud that his surname was spelt with a second 'a' instead of an 'e' so that it would be just like 'Laura' with an extra 'l' at the end.

It's always good to discover new diabetic role models. While we don't rejoice in others' misfortune, I've told Laura since her diagnosis at the age of 3 that diabetes won't stop her doing anything she wants to in this life, so it's good to find examples of high achievers with Type 1 diabetes. However, I may have overplayed this point: she once showed me in a guide to adult education classes a picture of a lady doing an extraordinary gymnastic feat, saying "I think she must be diabetic, because you said diabetics can do anything".

Laura loves old comedy films. Having watched Laurel and Hardy's complete works, she's now working her way through the Marx Brothers' oeuvre. Doting mother that I am, I wonder sometimes whether, with her precocious sense of humour and her clever way with words, she will one day be a comedy writer or performer herself.

If that's what she wants to be, Type 1 diabetes won't stop her. But had Laura been born in the era of silent movies, she wouldn't have had the chance to try. If diagnosed before 1922, she'd have been dead within weeks.

The early silent films we have been watching predate the discovery of insulin and the development of insulin therapy. (Stan Laurel became diabetic in the 1940s.) Even now, insulin doesn't cure Type 1 diabetes – it just holds it at bay. Without her daily insulin, Laura would simply die.

What we still need, so badly, is a cure. Then maybe, just maybe, one day, if Laura's name is up in lights as the twenty-first century's answer to Laurel and Hardy, her biographer, unlike Stan Laurel's, won't need to mention her diabetes. If we can raise enough funding, we can vanquish this terrible condition. We can edit Type 1 diabetes out of our lives and leave it, forgotten, on the cutting room floor.

If we can dream it, we can do it.

Let's do it.

~ 6 ~

RUN, RABBIT, RUN
(24 January 2014)

Before I had Laura, I flirted with the odd recreational run. After her diagnosis with Type 1 diabetes, I realised that running could be great therapy for me for the stress that arose from dealing with a chronically ill child. It allowed for some meditative me-time. What's more, taking part in sponsored runs provided a constructive opportunity to collect money to help fund research. It was also a good way to raise awareness of the cause.

I wrote this post and the following two in the year that I ran the Bristol 10K for JDRF.

January 1 is a rotten time to make New Year's Resolutions. The excitement of Christmas is over, the decorations are losing their charm, and the mornings and evenings seem darker than ever. Relentless advertising for the post-Christmas sales rubs in the fact that it's an awfully long time till payday. It's no wonder that January 24 is officially designated the most depressing day of the year.

This January brought only two sources of cheer: the opportunity to write cheques with cool dates (1/1/11 and 11/1/11) and, big kid that I am, my birthday. So this year I decided to be realistic about New Year's Resolutions: I resolved not to make any.

But then, a few weeks into the New Year, something wonderful happened: I looked up into the sky at 5pm and realised it was not entirely dark. A tiny tinge of blue still hovered behind the impending night sky, a promise of the spring to come. It was enough to make my personal sap rise. Then I spotted in my diary the fact that we were on the brink of Chinese New Year. Coming up was the Year of the Rabbit, so it wasn't too late for New Year's Resolutions after all!

Before I knew it, I found myself signing up to run the Bristol 10K. A leaner, faster, fitter new me would be just around the corner of 2011.

But it wouldn't be only me that benefited. I'd be fundraising for the Juvenile Diabetes Research Foundation. Every £60 I raised would pay for an hour of research to find a cure for Type 1 diabetes.

This horrible disease has blighted the life of my husband and my small daughter. Decades of research have made it possible for them at least to stay alive with Type 1 diabetes, provided they submit to daily invasive medical intervention. But what they, and millions of others, really want is for research to find a way to let them live without it. At present, there is no cure.

So, with my resolve strengthening as the daylight hours are lengthening, I have signed on the dotted line for the 10km charity run. I just wish I had a Chinese bank account, because then, when I write the deposit cheque, I could take enormous pleasure in dating it for the first day of the Chinese New Year: Rabbits Rabbits Rabbits/Rabbit.

WHAT WOULD IT TAKE
TO MAKE YOU RUN 10KM?
(1 January 2011)

Most of us will go through life never having run further than a few laps of the school field, usually under protest. But what would it take to make you run 10km?

- Advance warning that you're standing next to a ticking time bomb whose debris will fall within a 9.9999km radius?
- A race to pick up a jackpot-winning lottery ticket that you know is lying under a stone 10km away?
- A fast-moving forest fire that is chasing you towards a river 10km distant?

This may strike you as a hypothetical question – a bit like the old playground favourite "would you rather run a mile, jump a stile or eat a country pancake?" I remember, in my unathletic childhood aged about 8, falling for that one and choosing the country pancake, to the mirth of my interrogator who revealed that "country pancake" is rural slang for cowpat. (I must say that since I've been living in the country, I have never heard it referred to as such, though I still wouldn't choose a pancake from a country pub dessert menu, just in case.)

Everybody has some cause close to their heart, and I know I've found mine. In 6 weeks' time, I'll be running 10km in aid of JDRF.

My daughter was diagnosed with Type 1 diabetes at the age of 3, and that day our lives changed for ever. Gone were the blissful days of being able to eat what she liked, when she liked.

Gone were the low-maintenance days of being able to travel everywhere with a small handbag, uncluttered with hypodermics and hypo remedies. (I'd only just got rid of the nappy bag, too.)

Gone were the carefree days of visiting hospital only for the usual childhood A&E trips. Getting a doll's shoe stuck up her nose, as she did when she was 2, was a piece of cake compared to the unmissable daily routine of blood tests and injections. Such ailments don't put you at risk of serious long-term complications either, other than perhaps a fear of tiny footwear and long-handled tweezers.

For now, there is no cure for Type 1 diabetes. We're stuck with the daily inconvenience, pain and stress of treating the symptoms, and the long-term angst about the eventual effects on her health. It has got easier with time: at least she no longer hides under the kitchen table and sits on her hands when we're trying to prick her fingers for the blood tests. But there could be a cure, if enough money were thrown at the problem. There are many extraordinarily gifted and imaginative scientists poised to take their research on to the next step, if only funds permit.

If I could cure this terrible disease just by running, what a strange world that would be. But if that were the case, I'd run and run, and never stop till I reached the cure.

Running the Bristol 10K – and the sponsorship I might raise and the publicity I can attract – will be only a baby-step along the road to a permanent solution, but it beats eating a country pancake any day.

~ 8 ~

THE BEST REASON TO RUN
(15 May 2011)

While running the Bristol 10K this morning (she says casually), I was moved by the many charity T-shirts in evidence along the way. Runners were promoting many fabulous causes, from the well-known local hospice to obscure causes that I'd never even heard of, though I'll know them next time, thanks to those runners' efforts.

I love to run, but like many naturally unathletic latecomers to the running bug, I need a reason to run. A race date in my diary to train for and a formal commitment to a charity are both essential components to keep me piling up the miles.

My chosen charity, as evidenced by my running vest, was, unsurprisingly, JDRF. When I wavered in my training, my sense of obligation to early sponsors kept me at it. (Aaren Purcell and Bill Chapman, you were the leaders in that race, and I thought of you both on every training run.)

For people who are naturally athletic, running may be enough incentive in itself. What keeps them going is the constant striving for a new personal best, the new medal to add to their collection, the smart new race finisher T-shirt to boost their wardrobe of running clothes. Running to them is as blogging is to me: it's my favourite hobby, and I wouldn't dream of asking anyone to pay me for it.

But to me, no matter how fulfilling the run, it's a hugely wasted opportunity if you choose to trek round the route in a top that advertises only your favourite sportswear manufacturer or shows off your last year's holiday destination. Without a charity emblazoned on it, the runner's chest is a wasted opportunity, an empty billboard, a bare bus-shelter. There are plenty of charities who will be grateful if you fly their flag to raise awareness, even if you're not able to muster a bit of sponsorship. This simple effortless act could persuade wavering donors to stump up some cash next time they are asked by that charity. The crowd will cheer you on all the more because of it, and if they also thrust money into your hand for the cause along the route, so much the better.

So, if you're a runner without a cause, share mine: JDRF. And with every step you run, you'll be bringing the cure for Type 1 diabetes that little bit closer to the finishing line.

DIABETES IS ALWAYS WITH US
(27 August 2011)

We try not to let diabetes prevent our family from doing anything we want to do, and this includes foreign travel. We take to the road in our camper van at every opportunity, exploring new places and enjoying old favourites.

An important part of our preparation for any journey is to pack the right supplies to keep Gordon and Laura safe and well. More than once we've been grateful to a pharmacist in a foreign country when we've run out of a particular item in our kit – hypodermic needles, blood glucose test strips, even insulin. We once managed to lose a whole test kit on a school trip to France, requiring me to sprint to a Guernsey chemist's shop near the ferry port for a replacement moments before our ferry sailed.

Wherever we go, we carry the baggage of diabetes with us both literally and figuratively. I wrote the following piece after a month-long tour of France, when a trip to a museum reminded me once more why we really need to find a cure for Type 1 diabetes.

Pottering south from Dunkerque on our French odyssey this summer, we take the opportunity to revisit a memorable tourist attraction near St Omer.

La Coupole is a remarkable structure: a domed semi-underground cavern that would serve well as a film set for the lair of a James Bond villain. But it was the real life setting of a far greater horror. It's a Nazi military bunker, built to house and launch the revolutionary V2 bombs on London.

The museum has a particular significance for me. The London suburb in which I spent my childhood was a target for V2 bombs. I remember my grandma telling me that the most frightening thing about them was when they went silent: that meant they were about to hit the ground.

My 8-year-old daughter Laura has just finished a school topic about World War II. She and her classmates enjoyed it so much that they did not want the term to end. We're hoping the museum will complement her topic nicely, but I quickly realise that its displays are more horrific than I had remembered.

Fortunately some of the significance goes over Laura's head. She laughs at the spectacle of a slide show projected on a pocked and pitted rough brick wall, thinking it makes a funny cinema screen. It's actually a reconstruction of a firing squad's wall against which many French citizens met their death. She looks askance at a coarse stripey suit in a glass case: it offends her developing sense of fashion. I don't want to explain that someone may have died in this suit: it's the uniform of a concentration camp prisoner.

Watching films of French refugees heading south on foot, pushing sparse possessions in handcarts and wheelbarrows, I wonder what it would have been like if we'd been part of that procession. What would Laura have wanted to take with her? She's not good at travelling light. Seven cuddly toys have somehow stowed away in the camper van this holiday, although I'd told her to bring only two.

Then I remember an assignment she did at school. Her class had to plan what they'd have taken in their suitcases, had they been evacuees. No doubt many of them will have included modern luxuries such as iPods and XBoxes. Not so Laura. She thoughtfully stowed her favourite cuddly toy (so she'd have something to comfort her at night), a notebook and pen (in case she got bored), and her diabetes test kit. She drew a neat and accurate illustration of the lancets, test strips, and a blood glucose monitor that we use many times a day to manage her Type 1 diabetes.

I realise with a start that to have been among those French refugees would almost certainly have sentenced Laura to death, not from Nazi atrocities, but from her diabetes. Her complex medical needs, such as refrigeration for her insulin and supplies for her high-tech insulin pump, could never have been met on such a journey.

Suddenly Gordon and I find ourselves making excuses to leave the museum before Laura is ready to go. As we march across the car park back to the safety of our camper van, I hug my daughter a little tighter, patting the test kit in my handbag for reassurance. La Coupole is indeed an extraordinary monument, but as it recedes into the shadows behind us, I do not for a moment glance back.

~ 10 ~

WHAT I LIVE FOR
(10 May 2013)

My Buddhist author friend Satya Robyn invited me to take part in a mass blogging campaign on the day that, by chance, marked the sixth anniversary of Laura's diagnosis. Its theme was "What I Live For". Satya's campaign called for people all over the world to define on that day exactly what gave their lives meaning. Here is my contribution.

Not long after the turn of the millennium, my elderly neighbour James, aged 96, announced from his hospital bed: "This week, I shall decide whether or not I shall go on living."

A few months before, his wife Hester had died in a residential home where she'd been staying for a few days during his previous hospital treatment. They could just about manage to live at home together, but neither could cope alone.

Hester's death had been unexpected – well, as unexpected as it could be for a 90-year-old. She'd had breast cancer for several years, but in old age cancer grows slowly, and it was not cancer that killed her, but heart failure. One day she just sat on her bed, and as she fell back, her heart stopped.

James, bereft, was consoled that they'd achieved their goal of reaching their Silver Wedding anniversary. Only silver at their age? Yes, that's right. Childhood sweethearts, they'd been forbidden by their family to marry because they were first cousins. Disappointed, James eventually married someone else, but decades later, after his first wife had died, they decided to elope. Early one morning, these two old-age pensioners headed down the hill for a secret wedding in the parish church before anyone could stop them. They returned determined to do their best to live happily ever after.

During the final years of their marriage, they'd been taking turns to go in and out of hospital, like the little people in a weather house. Whenever they were too weak to visit each other, I was commissioned to ferry letters between them. Hester's eyesight was dim, so she'd ask me to read the messages aloud. This had to be done in a loud voice so that she could hear them properly. Invariably opening with old-fashioned terms of endearment ("Treasure…" was my favourite), these love letters – for that is what they were – made the whole ward smile.

To be honest, it probably wasn't a matter of choice whether James lived or died. He was 96 after all, and had recently been diagnosed with lung cancer. Like Hester's illness, it had been lurking for some time. That winter they'd become dramatically frailer. Most poignant was James's phone call to me on Boxing Day 1999, asking me to come round to plump up Hester's pillows as he didn't have enough strength. At this point, I was also nursing my first husband, who died of leukaemia ten days into the new millennium, just five days before Hester.

But don't feel sorry for me. I have never felt as loved as I did then. My family, friends and neighbours were unstinting in their support. I spent New Year's Eve at my husband's hospital bedside, before sleeping over at my parents' house nearby. I'd been dreading returning home next morning, until I found two candle lanterns on my windowsill, left by neighbours, one for each of us. It was a gift of hope.

Unlike James, I never doubted that I should go on living. After all, I was a child compared to him. I was just 39. Ever the optimist, ever the opportunist, after my first husband died I rebuilt my life. I remarried a couple of years later and, to everyone's surprise and delight, at the age of 43 I produced a daughter, Laura.

But it wasn't only this good fortune that gave me a reason to go on living. A further twist of fate lay in store. Just 13 days before my precious daughter's fourth birthday, she was rushed to hospital with Type 1 diabetes. If not caught and treated in time, it would have been fatal. We were lucky: we caught it early, and she survived, but it is a chronic incurable illness that will need daily medical intervention and vigilance for the rest of her life, unless a cure is found. (That's why I support JDRF, the charity dedicated to finding that cure.)

I remember with perfect clarity receiving the diagnosis. We sat in the office of Dr Mather, a lovely, gentle, kind lady GP who listened with increasing gravity to the symptoms before taking a tiny blood sample to test Laura's blood glucose.

"I wouldn't do a blood test on a child unless it was essential," she assured us. She looked at the test meter and was silent for a moment before announcing the result.

"It's 20."

We knew that the target range in a healthy person is between four and seven. We knew there was only one explanation.

On that 20 mile trip to A&E, where they were waiting poised to receive us as an emergency, I realised that our lives had changed forever. Ever since, my prime reason for living has been to keep my beautiful daughter healthy – to manage her condition to the best of my ability until she is old enough to take care of it herself.

But who am I kidding? Will I ever stop worrying about her well-being? I'm sure most mothers wouldn't, even without the diabetes. I'm sure I never will, even if I live to be as old as James. And I've just realised that if I *do* live to be as old as James, then Laura will be exactly the same age as I am now. This strikes me as a good omen, I don't know why.

It's also an extraordinary coincidence that Satya Robyn's "What I Live For" event falls precisely on the sixth anniversary of Laura's diagnosis with Type 1 diabetes. When I realised this, I knew I had to take part, to celebrate not the diabetes, but the daughter that I live for.

I'm very blessed.

SO HERE'S TO YOU, FREDERICK BANTING
(World Diabetes Day 2012)

On World Diabetes Day, let's not dwell on the trauma and heartache of the millions of people surviving around the world with Type 1 diabetes.

There's no point blaming them or anyone else, because it's a disorder that occurs through no fault of their own. They can't help the fact that diabetes changes their lives forever – and not in a good way. They'd rather not have to submit to the multiple daily blood tests and insulin injections or infusions. It's not such a big thing to make a fuss about – all they're trying to do is stay alive. Oh, and ward off the complications that can occur from badly controlled diabetes. It's a long list, it's dull and it's not pretty: blindness, amputation, premature heart disease. Oh, and I almost forgot the biggest one: death. Almost immediate death is inevitable for those not lucky enough to have access to modern diabetes management therapy. Better not to talk about it.

And anyway, it's not as if Type 1 diabetes is a new or original story: it's been around for centuries. It's just that before Sir Frederick Banting identified and isolated insulin in 1922, death would have been imminent for anyone unfortunate enough to develop the disease. There wouldn't have been as many Type 1 diabetics around as there are today. Well, not for long, anyway.

Nor is it something that matters only today, on World Diabetes Day, because for those who have Type 1 diabetes, every day is Diabetes Day. There's no day off. They'll have it for the rest of their lives, so why all the fuss today?

It's because today is Sir Frederick Banting's birthday. Happy birthday, Sir Frederick! Let's hope that some day soon, scientists will take your revolutionary life-saving work to the next level and make Type 1 diabetes history. I'm sure we've all got better ways to spend November 14. So let's make light of it instead. How about a song? Here's one to sing in celebration of the extraordinary pioneering work of Sir Frederick Banting, his Nobel-prize-winning research which made that magical substance, insulin, available today for therapy. It's not a cure, but it allows Type 1 diabetics to stay alive. Sir Frederick was not a materialistic man, selling the patent for insulin for just one Canadian dollar so that everyone could benefit. Modern drugs manufacturers, please take note.

Not surprisingly, Sir Frederick told me he doesn't want any birthday presents. Just send money to JDRF instead, because he couldn't wish for a better present than a cure.

And now let's finish with that song, to be sung to the tune of "Mrs Robinson", with apologies to Simon and Garfunkel:

And here's to Sir Frederick Banting,
Diabetics love you more than you can know (Wo, wo, wo)
God bless you, Sir Frederick Banting
At least since your research we've had a way
Alive to stay… hey, hey, hey

We'd like to celebrate the many lives that you have saved
We'd like to thank you for your research
Look around you, all you see are grateful patients' eyes
That Nobel prize was the very least that you deserved

And here's to Sir Frederick Banting
Diabetics love you even when hypo (Wo, wo, wo)
God bless you, Sir Frederick Banting
Your insulin injections help us stay
Alive today… hey hey hey

(Hide your syringe in a place where no one ever goes
Put it in your pantry with your dextrose
It's a little secret, just our T1D affair
Most of all, hide complications from the kids)

Coo coo ca choo, Frederick Banting
Diabetics love you more than you can know (Wo, wo, wo)
God bless you, Sir Frederick Banting
We wish that we could meet you just to say
Thanks to you, we're alive today

(Sitting on a sofa on a Sunday afternoon
Counting out the carbs before our dinner
Cry about it, shout about it
We don't get to choose
Every way we look at it, we lose)

Though now it's gone, our old carefree life,
Still we turn our grateful eyes to you (Woo, woo, woo)
For thanks to Sir Frederick Banting
Though normal life has left and gone away
Thanks to you, we're here to stay

APPEAL ON BEHALF OF JDRF

This book was published to mark World Diabetes Day 2014, but for people with Type 1 diabetes, every day is Diabetes Day. There will be no day off from diabetes until a cure is found. If you would like to help hasten the arrival of that glorious day, please donate £5, $5 or whatever you can spare to JDRF via their website: *www.jdrf.org.uk*.

JDRF is a registered charity in England and Wales number 295716 and in Scotland number SC040123.

ACKNOWLEDGEMENTS

Huge and heartfelt thanks to the lovely people who helped me prepare this book: Justin Webb for his eloquent foreword; Helen Hart and her team at SilverWood Books for expert advice and cover design; George Gooding for the new cover image of Laura; and Alison Jack for editing and proofreading.

Thanks also to my friends Jo Dury, Jacky Taylor, Lisa Hirst, Louise Arnold, Justine Daniels and Vicky Pember for pre-publication feedback; to Joanne Phillips and Shirley Wright for beta reading the first edition; author friends Dan Holloway, Judith Barrow and Satya Robyn for inspiration; and especially to Dr Carol Cooper for her support and encouragement to bring this book to a wider audience.

For keeping Laura and Gordon healthy and me sane, I am forever grateful to our National Health Service, in particular the Paediatric Diabetes team at the United Bristol NHS Trust and the Adult Diabetes team at the North Wiltshire NHS Trust. I will never forget the skill and compassion of Dr Mather, the GP who not only diagnosed Laura's condition but who also phoned a message through to us in hospital that evening, sending us her love. The NHS is truly wonderful.

Thanks also to my parents for their unswerving faith and support.

And finally, thanks to Laura and Gordon, for allowing me to write publicly about their condition for the benefit of others.

Debbie Young
World Diabetes Day 2014

ABOUT THE AUTHOR

After a long career in journalism, public relations and marketing, Debbie Young now lives and works in a small village in the Gloucestershire Cotswolds, where she and her Scottish husband Gordon and their daughter Laura are very involved in their local community.

She also enjoys travelling in the family's small motorhome, gaining inspiration wherever she goes for her wide-ranging blog.

She writes both fiction and non-fiction books and contributes regular columns to various magazines and websites. She is currently writing her first novel.

She is very active in the international self-publishing community. Commissioning Editor of the Alliance of Independent Authors' advice blog, she also helps other independent authors to market their books.

She is a public speaker for the JDRF and a member of its regional development committee. She is also a keen supporter of the UK children's charity Read for Good, whose Readathon sponsored reading programme encourages children to read for pleasure, and whose ReadWell scheme makes life better for seriously ill children in hospital by providing free books and storytellers.

She is never bored.

For more information about visit her website: www.authordebbieyoung.com
or follow her on Twitter: @DebbieYoungBN

OTHER BOOKS BY DEBBIE YOUNG

FICTION

Quick Change
The Owl & The Turkey
Stocking Fillers

NON-FICTION

Sell Your Books!
Opening Up To Indie Authors
(with Dan Holloway)

To join Debbie Young's mailing list
for news of new titles and events,
visit her website
www.authordebbieyoung.com

Printed in Great Britain
by Amazon

42525216R00025